Tania is an International, Multi-Award Winning Clinical Hypnotherapist and Psychotherapist supporting people with anxiety and related conditions across the world via Zoom, and in her private clinic in the heart of the Pennines, in Rochdale, UK.

She runs a monthly deep relaxation hypnotherapy group in Rochdale, and has affordable online memberships and workshops.

Tania is a Senior Lecturer for her business; 'Tania Taylor Hypnotherapy & Psychotherapy', and also Lectures on behalf of the 'Clinical Hypnotherapy School', who provide post qualification training to qualified hypnotherapists using the Solution Focused approach.

Tania continues to volunteer delivering free Hypnotherapy for local Macmillan events, and in her Facebook group weekly, helping people across the globe. She's always looking to help more people and welcomes you to join the Calm Your Mind group and to invite your family and friends too.

www.facebook.com/groups/
CalmYourMindFree

Tania Taylor

Sparkling Moments

30 Days of amazing

100% natural ways to boost
your feel-good brain chemicals

Published in 2019

ISBN: 978-1-9164514-4-5

Front cover and text design by Fuzzy Flamingo
www.fuzzyflamingo.co.uk

A catalogue for this book is available from the British Library.

For my beautiful family. I'm so lucky to have such a special group of people in my life, Adam, Chloe, and Callum. Thank you for all your support, love, and encouragement, and for reminding me I don't have to be superwoman, just me.

I love you all.

The wonderful truth about this book is that every page contains creative ideas for putting a bit of amazing back into your life. Whether you want to use it yourself, or gift it to a friend who needs a lift, this book will be sure to get those feel-good hormones and chemicals flowing through your system completely naturally.

DAY 1:

Make a Difference

Texting a friend or family member, giving way to a car ahead, holding the door open, or smiling in the queue at the supermarket. These are all wonderful ways to make a positive difference to the lives of others, which in turn makes you feel wonderful too.

Maybe this is something you already do. Can you keep track today of how often you do it? Can you look out for more opportunities where you might not usually make a difference?

At the end of the day, reflect on all the people you have made a difference to. Allow yourself to smile or even laugh as you think about the amazing moments you created today for others.

DAY 2:

Wake up to Happy Thoughts

Easier said than done, right? You might have had a bad dream, you might not want to get out of bed, or maybe your stress bucket is overflowing with stress right now.

So, let's find ways to make it happen.

Step 1: Decide on a happy thought you would like to wake up to. If you could wake up to any happy thought you could possibly think of, what would it be?

Step 2: Do something that is going to remind you of it when you first wake up. Maybe it's your phone screensaver. Maybe it's a Post-it note on the mirror. Maybe it's a picture or a clipping from a magazine. Whatever it is, pop it somewhere you will notice it as soon as you wake up.

DAY 3:

Enjoy Your Surroundings

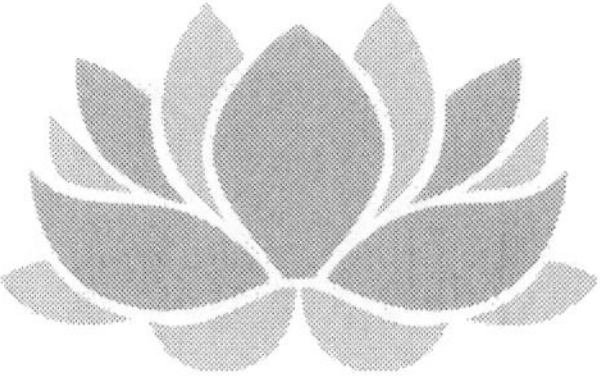

Look around you right at this very moment. Find three items that you are pleased to have.

Spend a moment thinking about why you are pleased to have each item.

Do any of them have a funny memory linked to them?

Every time you eat today, look for three more items wherever you are.

DAY 4:

Being Kind to You

Looking after our self is often something we put at the bottom of our to-do lists. So, what could you squeeze in today that would feel like you were giving yourself some well-deserved 'me time'?

There are a few ideas below:

Netflix, cinema, brunch, lunch, dinner, gym, swimming, visit friends, spend time with your partner, with your family, have a long bath, book a massage, start reading a book, sit in the garden.

DAY 5:

You Are Strong

Think back over the last few years. How many challenges have you overcome? How many battles have you faced and survived?

What about this week? How many mini triumphs have you had?

Maybe you got out of bed on time every day. Maybe you made a home cooked meal. Maybe you met a deadline or finally got around to calling up a friend?

Did you congratulate yourself?

What did you reward yourself with?

Every day you face lots of challenges, and every day of your life so far has seen you overcome every hurdle.

Today, celebrate the hurdles you have jumped, reward yourself with something special just for you.

Tip: Reward doesn't have to be food and drink. Reward can be looking in the mirror and congratulating yourself, treating yourself to a pamper in the bath, treating yourself to some time to spend reading.

DAY 6:

Loving You

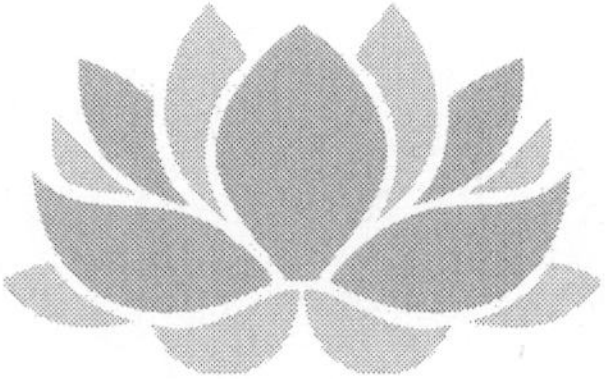

Think of a small child, a toddler. What happens when they see themselves in a mirror? Do they laugh and play? Clap their hands? Dance? Smile?

Now consider you as you were at the same age. Imagine yourself looking in the mirror. Smile at yourself. Enjoy the wonderful way you pay attention to yourself without judgement, without worry or fear, enjoy loving being you.

Every time you look in the mirror today, imagine being you as a toddler and smiling at yourself with the same love and admiration as you did when you were so much younger. Say to yourself:

You are amazing!

DAY 7:

Planning Ahead

Today is all about planning for the future. When we plan something to look forward to, simply looking forward to the event boosts our feel-good hormones.

So, let's take a moment to consider between one and three activities you like to do. Maybe it's a walk? Or a phone call with a friend you haven't spoken to in a while? Maybe it's a yoga class?

Whatever it is, spend some time today setting these events in motion. Get them in your diary and enjoy that feeling of accomplishment.

Look forward to your lovely plans.

DAY 8:

Coping Better with Stressful Events

Some days will be stressful. Sometimes, we are thrown a curveball and our day doesn't go how we planned.

Today is focused on what we can do to prepare for stressful events.

First, let's imagine that there is a scale to each day. Each day you move up and down the scale. 10/10 is the best you could possibly feel and 0/10 is the opposite.

When we're feeling a 10/10 something stressful might occur, but we find ourselves coping so much better because we were already feeling good.

Think about the last response you had to something stressful.

Is it exactly how you would like to respond if something similar occurs in future? Or would you have felt better if you had responded slightly differently?

Maybe, a different response would have helped you cope better with the situation?

Today it's time to prepare an ideal response to stressful situations. We know we can't change the external world, but we can change our response to it to ensure that we cope better with any challenges life throws our way.

DAY 9:

I Love You

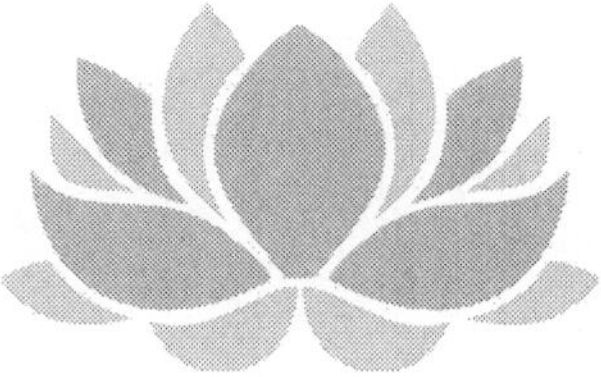

When was the last time you told someone that you love them?

Consider all the people in your life you love.

Do they know you love them?

Today's task is sending a simple text to all the people you love. An example is below:

> Hi, it's me. I'm just sending you a little text to let you know I care about you, and I'm so grateful to have you in my life. I love you. X

Enjoy reading your responses and feel good about having special people in your life. Don't forget to send one to yourself!

DAY 10:

Good Qualities

Think of a boss, a colleague, or maybe a teacher in your life whom you thought was great.

Write down all their good qualities.

Now spend some time considering the good qualities they would write down about you.

All those qualities you see in others, and that you believe others see in you, are all qualities you do have yourself. We often can only see the good qualities in others that we also hold ourselves.

DAY 11:

Flying Dinosaurs and Cute Bunnies

If I asked you to write a list of all the behaviour habits that you don't want to do anymore, I'm sure you'd be able to come up with some.

However, that's NOT what I'm going to ask you to do today.

Instead, I have a more difficult task for you. I'd like you to consider something you want to stop doing, and then focus on what you would like to do instead. What can you replace it with?

If I said to you: 'Don't think about flying dinosaurs,' you WILL think about flying dinosaurs. If I say: 'Think about a cute bunny,' you will think about a cute bunny. Our brain needs a focus and a destination: If you don't want to do something or think something anymore, you must have something you want to do instead so that your brain can stop focusing on what you don't want to do.

So, what are you going to replace your unwanted habit with today?

DAY 12:

Overcoming Our Negative Bias

Did you know that we are hardwired to think negatively?

It is a survival mechanism. If we worry about something that might cause us harm in the future, we are less likely to go ahead and do it, which means human race survival on a global scale. However, this negative bias was made for us back in the cave man/woman days. It prevented us from jumping off cliffs to certain death.

Today, we don't need to use the negative bias with everything we do because the perceived danger isn't always life threatening.

So, today it's time to consider what has

been playing on your mind recently. What is it you have spent a little bit of time worrying about, and how is it life threatening to you?

Your most likely answer here is that it's certainly not life threatening for you. So, let's instead look at the same scenario you have been worrying about using your positive frame of mind instead. Put pen to paper and write down all the things that might go well. What would be the results if everything worked out perfectly? What difference would that make for you?

Now you have shown your negative bias that this is a safe situation and one that may result in rewards and gratitude instead.

DAY 13:

Shifting Your Focus

Unlucky for some? But not for all!

The number thirteen is only unlucky to those using their negative bias to search for bad luck surrounding that number. What if instead you spent the day focusing on all things that were good?

If anything goes wrong, that's okay, you don't need to focus your time or energy on that today because today you are giving your all to focus on nice moments, small moments, delicious food or drink moments, engaging conversation moments, beautiful smells moments, and all of the other moments in the day that enable you to feel rewarded, full of hope, and good in the moment.

DAY 14:

A Picture Paints a Thousand Words

So does a photo!

Today it's time to go through your day snapping pics of items that bring a smile to your face. Maybe you spot a beautiful flower, or perhaps a cute animal. Maybe you're by the ocean or a forest. Maybe there's a little bird hopping along a branch nearby. Or maybe that tree you walk past every day just looks more interesting today. Maybe it's the food on your plate, or your new clothes.

Whatever it is, studies have shown that taking pictures in this way every day for three weeks rewires your brain into coping better with life's challenges and rating yourself higher on questionnaires about how good you feel.

DAY 15:

Time to Look After You and Your Sleep

Our body does so much whilst we are sleeping, particularly in our brain. Sleep is essential for good mental health. So, if we're having lots of difficulties with sleeping then it's important to look at our habits around going to sleep.

If we allow that negative bias to tell us we won't sleep tonight, then we will struggle to sleep. If we take time to put some new habits in place to help us sleep better, then we will sleep better.

There's one thing on your mind already that you know if you changed you might find it a little easier to relax and unwind before bed. Maybe it's your screen time. Maybe it's something else. Take one step at a time and slowly but surely introduce a new routine to your evenings.

Tip: Our body won't produce melatonin, which helps us prepare for sleep, if we're having a certain light emitted from our screen devices. The 'blue' light emitted means melatonin won't start being produced until we get into bed, so it will take us much longer to get to sleep. Some phones now have the option to turn the 'blue light' off, take a look at your settings.

Tip: Listen to my hypnotherapy when you're going to sleep – search for me on YouTube – Tania Taylor Hypnotherapy.

DAY 16:

Feeling All of Our Feelings

Being happy all the time is an unrealistic expectation. It's a goal you're aiming for that is sure to see you fail.

Why?

Because we're human, and we can't control external factors, we can only control our response to them.

It is important to recognise that you are allowed to feel all your feelings. However, when we are feeling particularly low or anxious, we may decide that this isn't how we want to feel forever and so we can do something as simple as marking a date in the diary that is intended to be the date that we will begin taking care of ourselves again.

Setting a date gives us time to acknowledge that we want to feel the way we are doing right now, whilst recognising that it isn't how we want to feel forever. It also gives us time to build our confidence in making a change to our current circumstances. Maybe we will plan to meet up with some friends or get out of bed and get dressed that day. Maybe we will plan a relaxing bath or to watch something uplifting on television such as a comedy.

DAY 17:

Making Your Day Special

How? However you want to and within the resources you have that are yours.

Imagine if today really was a special day. A day that you've experienced in the past that was particularly special for you. Think of all those wonderful emotions you felt on your special day.

Did you find yourself smiling more, perhaps? Maybe your movements were slightly different when you walked. Maybe your shoulders were back, and your head was held a little higher because you knew your day was special.

Spend today walking around like it's another

special day, even though it is a normal day for you. This is how you make any day special. Just by doing this you are getting wonderful natural boosts of hormones that make you feel your day is even more special and enjoyable.

Enjoy having a special day just because you can, just because you've decided that today WILL be special.

DAY 18:

And STOP

Set a little reminder to go off once an hour on your phone today.

Each time it goes off, do the following:

- STOP.
- Drop and relax your shoulders.
- Unclench your teeth.
- Relax your tongue from the roof of your mouth.
- Take three long deep breaths.

Notice how much more productive you are today.

DAY 19:

Your Month Ahead

Today let's look ahead to the following four weeks.

What would you like to achieve this month?

What is realistic? Have you created a plan or a little list?

Consider what your top five priorities are for this month.

They could be:

- Family time.
- Buying birthday gifts.
- Seeing friends.
- Going to the cinema.
- Walking more.

Whatever they are, jot them down on a

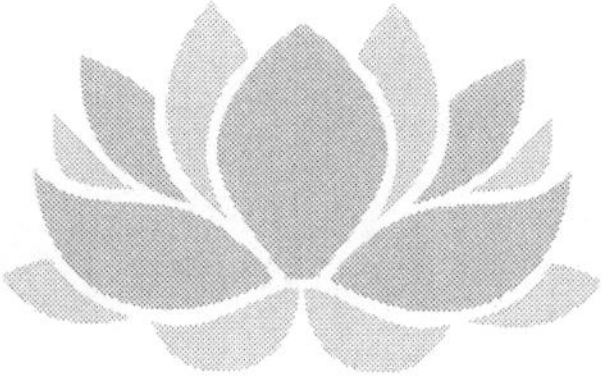

piece of paper, and next to each one plan a realistic and achievable timeframe for you to accomplish that particular task.

If it's a reoccurring task like going for a walk, set a day of the week or a time of the day when you know you will feel most motivated.

Then choose what the best reminder for you might be so that you are even more likely to carry out the task. It could be writing it on your wall calendar or putting a reminder on your Google Home or Alexa… or even a note by your bedside.

When we plan and visualise an achievable event, we store it as a safe and acceptable behaviour to use in the future and so we are much more likely to do what we want than if we don't plan ahead.

DAY 20:

The Joys of Reminders

Set a reminder for every hour today.

Each time your reminder goes off, consider the last hour and find at least one thing within the last hour that was good. No excuses.

At the end of your day, read your list of all the wonderful things that were good in your day, and notice just how great your day is, even when not everything goes the way you had anticipated.

DAY 21:

Mindful Eating

Every time you eat, spend some time considering what had to happen to get each item of food from where it began to here on your plate.

An example might be a carrot.

I wonder where that carrot was grown? Who planted it? Was it hand planted? Did a big machine plant it? Who was driving the machine? How long did it have to stay in the ground? Who picked it and how was it picked? Where did it go next? How long did it travel in the back of a lorry? Did it have to go through border control? Did it ever go through a factory of some kind? Who packaged it and took it to the supermarket or local grocery store? How many hands went in to making sure it got to you today?

When we use mindfulness regularly, we find ourselves coping so much better with life. When we use mindfulness with food there are all kinds of benefits. A quick Google search will tell you all about it.

DAY 22:

Reflection

It's time to look back at the challenges from your past. Everyone has some significant events that stand out for them as particularly difficult times.

One person's pain is not more significant than another's. Our perception of pain can differ from one person to the next, but also even our own perception of pain can differ from one day to the next, dependent on how resilient we are feeling at that time.

Each of the challenges you have just thought about are challenges you have overcome. You got through them. Some of them you may even wonder how you got through them at all, and yet, you DID get through them.

You have got through so much in your life, it's time to reflect today and acknowledge just how strong and powerful you are. It's time to take credit for your ability to endure pain and hardship because you have done, and you're here now doing the best that you can.

Today it's time to congratulate yourself on being amazing, because you are amazing.

DAY 23:

Touch

Did you know that TOUCH can have a profound impact on our ability to feel good? Touch can help lower our levels of cortisol (stress hormone) and increase our levels of oxytocin (feel good hormone).

- Is there someone's hand you can hold today?
- Or maybe someone you can get a reciprocal hug from?
- Do you have a pet you can fuss over?

A twenty-second hug or hand hold gives you a lovely little burst of oxytocin.

Give yourself some time to feel calmer, to touch, and enjoy being in the company of someone you care about today. Don't be afraid to give yourself a hug!

DAY 24:

Admiration

Think about someone you look up to. Someone you really admire.

Maybe they're in your life now, maybe it's someone from your past.

If they were walking in your shoes today, what would they do differently that you would admire about them?

Today you can take a few moments to consider if this is a quality you can introduce into your day today too.

DAY 25:

Smiling is Infectious

- Time to take a moment or two throughout your day to smile at someone you wouldn't normally smile at.
- To hold a door open you might not have held open before.
- To give a compliment to at least five people.

See what a difference you make to them, and what a difference it makes to you.

Don't worry if you're not thanked, or that smile is not reciprocated. We don't know what is going on in that person's life right now that means they might not have the confidence or be in the right frame of mind to return that smile or compliment, just feel at peace with the fact that you have added a sparkling moment to their very complicated day. Be proud of you.

DAY 26:

Random Act of Kindness

Kindness is a wonderful tool as long as we don't use it so much on others that it results in us forgetting to be kind to ourselves too. Today, let's take a look at some random acts of kindness you can do.

I've popped a few ideas below:

- A little thank you note to someone who needs it right now.
- Maybe you decide that today you'll take your neighbour's bins out for them.
- You could compliment a colleague or friend's work.
- Or perhaps you will compliment someone on an item of clothing they're wearing.

It can be absolutely anything that makes you feel good, because when we're being kind

to others, we activate a chemical hormone called oxytocin. The same feel-good chemicals we get when we stroke an animal, or give someone a hug.

Enjoy being kind to others today.

DAY 27:

Positive Affirmations

If you could say the most uplifting thing you could think of to yourself every day what would it be?

It might be ‘I can be amazing whenever I want to be’.

Or

‘I love who I am’.

Or

‘I am super fabulous and looking great today’!

Whatever it is, grab a Post-it note, write it down and stick it on the mirror you use most often.

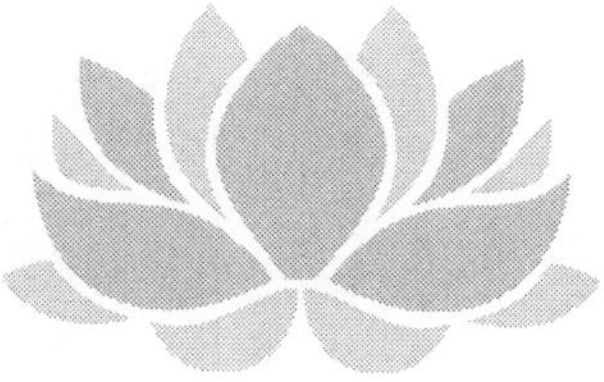

Congratulate yourself on being so fabulous! The more you tell yourself something, the more acceptable it becomes to your brain.

So, instead of looking at yourself in the mirror and berating you, it's time to look at yourself and tell yourself something kind.

DAY 28:

Utilising Your Love

Who do you love most in the world?

What do you love so much about them?

How do you help to nurture them and build their confidence and self-belief?

Write down your answers.

Now consider how much time and commitment you spend nurturing and building your own confidence. We can love ourselves just as much as we love our most special person in the world, if only we give ourselves permission to treat our self with such loving kindness.

How can you use those wonderfully transferable skills of loving and caring about someone else on yourself?

DAY 29:

Surrounding People with Love

Today you have a challenge.

A challenge to surround people with love.

It isn't about being "woo woo". Today is about acknowledging that some people are struggling to be as calm and collected as you, even if you're not feeling quite as calm and collected as you'd necessarily like to feel right now.

That driver that cuts you up on the motorway: instead of cursing, try surrounding them with love for a safe journey home.

The trolley that bashes yours in the supermarket: surround its owner with love for the rest of their shopping trip.

That driver might be rushing to hospital. That trolley owner might have coordination difficulties. When we are caught up in a moment, we can be very quick to jump to conclusions and make assumptions that are often not true. This results in us feeling angry or frustrated.

Stopping ourselves in our tracks, and instead considering the reasons this event may have happened and spending a moment just to hope that person is safe and well, can turn our ability to cope with challenging scenarios completely on its head. Notice how great you feel the next time you stop yourself being angry at a small event like the examples above.

DAY 30:

Sparkling Moments

What is a sparkling moment? It's a moment that feels amazing for you. By now you've had 30 days of amazing in your life. Think back over all of the amazing moments you have created all for yourself. Which was your sparkling moment? Which one really stood out for you?

At night when we get into bed, we can spend a moment or two considering what our sparkling moment of the day is.

It is a great way to engage the feel good chemicals that help us to relax right before we go to sleep. At the end of a week or a month, or even a year, you could even reflect back on which was your overall sparkling moment too.

Contact Me:

www.Tania-Taylor.co.uk

https://www.facebook.com/
TaniaTaylorHypnotherapy/

https://www.instagram.com/
taniataylorhypnotherapy/

Printed in Great Britain
by Amazon

34345774R00032